Feeding Your Baby Naturally From The Start

By.

Danna Davis

# Table Of Contents

## Breakfast & Purees

## Specialty Beverages

# Introduction

The purpose of this book is to educate parents on how to safely introduce natural/organic foods into their child's diet right from the start.
Store bought baby foods contain preservatives, sodium, and sugars that can potentially harm the baby especially at such an early age.

By utilizing simple inexpensive recipes we can start a revolution to get our children on the right path to eating healthy foods at an early age.
It is our hope that as an owner of this book, you will share these teachings with as many new or seasoned parents as you can.

Together we can raise healthy children and give back to our communities something so simple yet so vital, for many generations to come.

We hope you enjoy making these recipes, we know your baby will enjoy them too!

# Important

The information given here is meant as a guide and does not replace professional medical advice. Please discuss the introduction of any new foods or drinks with your baby's doctor.

Giving baby juice before 6 months of age

Both the American Academy of Pediatrics and the UK Foods Standards Agency state that you should not give your baby juice before he is at least 6 months of age.

Up to this stage, he/she is getting all the nutrients they needs for healthy growth and development from breast milk/formula. Feeding a baby juice can make them feel full and cause less tolerance for milk, which will deprive he/she of these essential nutrients.

# Breakfast & Purees

Organic Rice Cereal

Babies 6 – 12 months


1/4 c. (around 1 oz) brown rice powder
8 fl.oz. (1 c. ) water

Add milk of your choice (breast milk, soy, almond, coconut, rice, etc.)


To make the rice powder, grind brown rice in a blender or food processor. You can use white rice if you prefer, but this page explains why brown rice is more nutritious.

Bring the water to a boil.

Add the rice powder, stirring constantly with a wire whisk.

Reduce the heat to very low and simmer gently for about 10 minutes (don't forget to keep stirring, or the rice will stick).

Then stir in enough formula or breast milk to give the consistency that's best for your baby.

Once a baby has been introduced to fruit, you could always add a little of their favorite fruit puree for sweetness.

*Important benefits gained from eating brown rice include a reduced risk of type 2 diabetes and lower levels of cholesterol.
Enjoy!!!!!

Note: It is also important to introduce new foods one at a time, with at least three days in between to make sure your baby's not allergic.

Organic Baby Oatmeal

Babies 6 – 12 months

1/4 c. of ground oats (use regular or steel cut when possible), ground in blender or food processor

3/4 c. - 1 c. water or breast milk (for sweetness)

Bring liquid to boil in saucepan. Add the oatmeal powder while stirring constantly.  Simmer for 10 minutes, whisking constantly, mix in breast milk and fruits if desired. Serve warm!!! Oatmeal (one cup, regular, non-fortified & cooked) Protein - 5.94g

Note:
VITAMINS:
Vitamin A - 0 IU
Vitamin C - 0 mg
Vitamin B1 (thiamine) - .17 mg
Vitamin B2 (riboflavin) - .04 mg
Niacin - .53 mg
Folate - 14 mcg

Contains some other vitamins in small amounts.

MINERALS:
Potassium - 164 mg
Phosphorus - 162 mg
Magnesium - 84 mg
Calcium - 21 mg
Sodium - 9 mg
Iron - 2.11 mg
Selenium - 12 mg

Also contains small amounts of zinc, magnesium and copper.

Organic Barley Cereal

Babies 6 – 12 months

2 oz. (1/4 c.) ground barley*

12 fl. oz. (1 1/2 c.) water

1 tsp. Peaches

You can grind the barley in a food processor, or with a grain grinder. When grinding in small batches it will give gives a better result. Pour the water into a small saucepan and bring to the boil.

Add the powdered barley, stirring constantly. Bring back to the boil, then reduce the heat and simmer gently for around 15 to 20 mins. An alternative to grinding the barley is to simply cook it in the regular way, then place the cooked barley in a food processor and blend with enough formula to give the desired consistency.

However you cook it, stirring in some mashed peaches will sweeten the barley and you can also try mixing it with other fruit purees.  Serve & enjoy!!!!

Note:
1 teaspoon fruit, gradually increased to 1/4 to 1/2 cup in 2 or 3 feedings
1 teaspoon vegetables, gradually increased to 1/4 to 1/2 cup in 2 or 3 feedings
3 to 9 tablespoons cereal, in 2 or 3 feedings

Carrot Puree

Babies 6 – 12 months


5-6 carrots, peeled and cut into small chunks

Water (as needed)


Steam sliced carrots in a vegetable steamer for 20 minutes or until tender. Remove carrot from steamer and do not reserve the cooking liquid as Nitrates may seep into the cooking water.

Place carrot in a food processor; process until smooth.

Add water as necessary to achieve a smooth, thin consistency.

Refrigerate leftovers in BPA-free containers for up to 3 days. Freeze leftovers for up to 3 months. Thaw overnight in your refrigerator.

Green Peas Puree

Babies 6 – 12 months

Fresh or Frozen Peas (avoid canned peas)

Water (as needed)

Wash the Peas - If you decide to use frozen peas, skip this step and move to the next.

Place the peas in a steamer and cook for 3 to 5 minutes, or until tender. Drain peas and rinse with cold water for three minutes to stop the cooking process.

Puree or Mash the Peas
Puree peas in a blender until smooth.

Add water as needed to reach desired consistency.

Refrigerate leftovers in BPA-free containers for up to 3 days. Freeze leftovers for up to 3 months. Thaw overnight in your refrigerator.

Avocado Puree

Babies 6 – 12 months

1 fresh avocado

Water (as needed)

Omega-3-rich avocados are a great first introduction to solid foods.

Slice avocado down the middle, lengthwise, working around the pit. Twist each half of the avocado until it pulls apart. Use a spoon to pry out the pit, or stick the blade of a sharp knife into the pit and twist until the pit pops out. Cut slices lengthwise in the avocado just down to the skin and then scoop the flesh out of the avocado with a spoon.

Puree in a blender until smooth.

Add water as needed to reach desired consistency. For extra creaminess, puree the avocado with breast milk or formula instead of water.

Refrigerate leftovers in BPA-free containers for up to 3 days. Freeze leftovers for up to 3 months. Thaw overnight in your refrigerator.

Butternut Squash Puree

Babies 6 – 12 months

1 butternut squash

Water (as needed)

Cut butternut squash in half, scoop out seeds.

Place halves face down in a pan and cover with an inch of water.

Bake in a 400 degree oven for 40 minutes to 1 hour – be sure the "shell/skin" puckers and halves feel soft then scoop squash "meat" out of the shell.

Place squash "meat" into blender and begin pureeing.

Add water as necessary to achieve a smooth, thin consistency.

Refrigerate leftovers in BPA-free containers for up to 3 days. Freeze leftovers for up to 3 months. Thaw overnight in your refrigerator.

Apple Puree

Babies 6 – 12 months

2 eating apples (of your choice)

4 - 5 tbsp. water

Peel and chop the apples. Place into a heavy based saucepan with the water. Cover over a low heat for 6 to 8 minutes until tender.

Puree in a food processor or place in a bowl and use a hand blender.

Refrigerate leftovers in BPA-free containers for up to 3 days. Freeze leftovers for up to 3 months. Thaw overnight in your refrigerator.

Orange Puree

Babies 6 – 12 months

1 ripe orange (peeled, seeded and cut into chunks)

1 cup organic apple juice (or water)

Blend orange in blender until a smooth liquid.

Add organic apple juice (or water) to blender and further blend.

Refrigerate leftovers in BPA-free containers for up to 3 days. Freeze leftovers for up to 3 months. Thaw overnight in your refrigerator.

Strawberry Puree

Babies 6 – 12 months

6 whole strawberries

Water (as needed)

Wash strawberries with a mixture of three parts water and one part white vinegar to remove bacteria. Rinse under cool running water and dry. Remove stem and slice each strawberry in half, lengthwise, then into quarters.

Puree in a food processor or blender until smooth. Add water as needed to reach desired consistency.

For chunkier strawberry puree, which is ideal for babies 10 months or older, mash the strawberries with a potato masher instead of pureeing it.

Refrigerate leftovers in BPA-free containers for up to 3 days. Freeze leftovers for up to 3 months. Thaw overnight in your refrigerator.

Banana Puree

Babies 6 – 12 months

1 medium fresh banana (Choose bananas with blemish-free yellow peel)

Water or Breast milk (as needed)

Bananas have a smooth, squishy texture that's easy for babies to mash between their gums. They're an ideal first fruit after babies have tried several different kinds of veggies.

1 medium fresh banana mixed with formula or breast milk yields 6 to 8 ounces of puree.

Wash, Peel & Slice the Banana.

Puree blender until smooth. (Fresh banana has a light purple-brown color when pureed.) Add water or breast milk as needed to reach desired consistency. For extra creaminess, puree the banana with breast milk or formula instead of water.

Refrigerate leftovers in BPA-free containers for up to 3 days. Freeze leftovers for up to 3 months. Thaw overnight in your refrigerator.

Mango Puree

Babies 6 – 12 months


1 ripe mango

Water (as needed)


Wash the Mango; rinse under cool running water and dry.

Peel & Slice the Mango

Puree mango in a blender until smooth.

Add water as needed to reach desired consistency.

For chunkier mango puree, which is ideal for babies 10 months or older, mash the mango with a potato masher instead of pureeing it.

Refrigerate leftovers in BPA-free containers for up to 3 days. Freeze leftovers for up to 3 months. Thaw overnight in your refrigerator.

Plum Puree

Babies 6 – 12 months

1 whole, fresh plum

Water (as needed)

Wash the plum; rinse under cool running water and dry.

Boil Plum for 45 seconds and place into ice bath. Then, Peel the Plum

Slice plum in half, lengthwise, working your way around the pit. Slice each half into even-sized slices then quarter each slice.

Puree plum in a blender until smooth.

Add water as needed to reach desired consistency.

Refrigerate leftovers in BPA-free containers for up to 3 days. Freeze leftovers for up to 3 months. Thaw overnight in your refrigerator.

# Specialty Beverages

Organic Coconut Water

Babies 6 + months

2-3 tsp. coconut water and slowly increase the quantity

Coconut Water (as well as all other juices) should always be served to your baby in a cup, never a bottle.

Coconut water is a near perfect drink as it contains plenty of minerals like potassium, sodium, calcium, magnesium, iron, copper, phosphorus and Vitamins B complex and C.

Start with 2-3 teaspoons and slowly increase the quantity. Make sure you use a tender green coconut instead of those in which the skin has turned brown.

Coconut water is ideal in preventing dehydration, especially when children get diarrhea. It replenishes the natural salts lost by the body. In the hot summer months, when your toddler is thirsty, coconut water is much more beneficial than packaged fruit juices and aerated drinks which only contains empty calories.

Apple Juice

Babies 6 + months


1 cup chopped apples


1 cup water


Boil the chopped apples in water for about two minutes. Strain through a sieve. Serve cooled in summer or lukewarm in winter.

You can also add carrots to this recipe to get a delicious carrot and apple punch.

Apple juice (as well as all other juices) should always be served to your baby in a cup, never a bottle.

Keep in an airtight container in the refrigerator for 2-3 weeks

Grape Juice

Babies 6 – 12 months

2 cup grapes

5-6 cup water (needed)

Wash the grapes thoroughly, removing any stems or blemished fruit. Mash them with a spoon until juice begins to run out.

Remove the grapes from the stalk and place them in a blender.

Blend the grapes. You do not want them to be liquidized, just chopped up.

Place the blended grapes in a sieve over a bowl to drain off the juice.

Use a spoon to press down on the grape puree to extract every last bit of juice.

Grape juice (as well as all other juices) should always be served to your baby in a cup, never a bottle.

Carrot Juice

Babies 6 + months

1 medium sized organic carrot

Carrot juice (as well as all other juices) should always be served to your baby in a cup, never a bottle.

Carrots is one of the perfect first foods for your baby.

Sterilize all the utensils either using a sterilizer or by placing the utensils in boiling hot water.

Select a Medium sized carrot.
Peel the skin.

With a handy grater, grate the carrot. (a grater that has small holes is preferred)

After washing your hands with disinfectant, take the grated carrot in your palm, make a fist and squeeze the carrot so that the juice can be collected in a cup underneath.

Squeeze the juice out of the carrot until only the chaff remains

Keep in an airtight container in the refrigerator for 2-3 weeks

Chamomile Tea

Teas are suitable for (After 6 months)

1 chamomile teabag or 1 heaping teaspoon loose-leaf chamomile tea or dried chamomile flowers

2-3 oz. (about 250 ml) water, brought just to the boil

Add the teabag or loose-leaf tea to your favorite cup or mug.

Cool the just-boiled water slightly and then add to your baby's bottle.

Let your chamomile tea steep for 5 to 10 minutes

Remove the teabag or loose tea leaves.

Chamomile is known for its soothing and relaxing properties. It is used as a natural sleep aid. So not only will it sooth a gassy baby but help your baby relax. Babies need their sleep just as much as we do. This herb can help relax a inconsolable baby so both of you can be happy. If you need more help, see how I can help your baby sleep through the night!

Teething:
No need to use dangerous over the counter teething jells. The FDA issued a warning against the use of those products anyway. Chamomile is great for teething. Soak a clean washcloth in the tea and let your baby gnaw on it.

Mint Leaf Tea

Teas are suitable for (After 6 months)

1 mint teabag or 1 heaping teaspoon loose-leaf mint tea or dried mint leaves

2-3 oz. (about 250 ml) water, brought just to the boil

Add the teabag or loose-leaf tea to your favorite cup or mug.

Cool the just-boiled water slightly and then add to your baby's bottle.

Let your mint tea steep for 5 to 10 minutes

Remove the teabag or loose tea leaves.

IMPORTANT: The information given here is meant as a guide and does not replace professional medical advice. Please discuss the introduction of any new foods or drinks with your baby's doctor.

Giving baby juice before 6 months of age:

Both the American Academy of Pediatrics and the UK Foods Standards Agency state that you should not give your baby juice before he is at least 6 months of age.

Up to this stage, your baby is getting all the nutrients he needs for healthy growth and development from breast milk/formula. Feeding baby juice can make him feel full and cause him to accept less milk, which will deprive him of these essential nutrients